If you feel this booklet has been beneficial, I would ask that you pass it on to one whom you feel would also benefit from it. And ask them to do the same, and so on, and so on.

Charles Tindell

Life's Journey:

What's in your suitcase?

Dealing with the aging process?

Items one might consider to pack.

Lessons learned while working as a chaplain with those who have already made the journey.

Charles Tindell

Dedicated to those who have traveled before us

on the journey

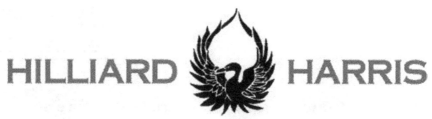

HILLIARD HARRIS

P.O. Box 84

Boonsboro, Maryland 21713-0084

Copyright © 2022

By Charles Tindell

First Edition—2022

ISBN-1-591333-483-7

ISBN-978-1-59133-483-5

Book Design: S. A. Reilly

Manufactured/Printed in the United States of America
2022

As a chaplain for thirteen years at a large long-term care facility, I learned a lot from the people I served.

In the following pages are some thoughts on what one might consider packing in a suitcase as one travels on life's journey. This is by no means an exhaustive list, but I would like to think if anyone packed these things, they would not only be better prepared to take on the journey, but would find that the traveling goes much easier and is more fulfilling.

A Positive Attitude

Are you the type of person who has a positive attitude about life? You may not like the things that happen along the journey of life but you decided to make the best of them. Would this describe you? Do you have this packed away in your suitcase for life's journey?

A gentleman who resided on the second floor of the long-term care facility I worked at had a stroke. Paralyzed on one side, he had no use of his right arm or leg. He was in a wheelchair. His speech, affected. His smile, crooked. Now, if you think that the poor guy stayed in his room all day long and felt sorry for himself, you would be wrong.

Whenever I went to find him in his room, he was gone. I discovered that he would be wheeling all over the facility using his good left arm and leg.

He would smile his crooked smile at other residents, staff, and visitors. People loved to see him.

Did he like that he was in a wheelchair and paralyzed on one side? Of course not. But he made the decision that no matter what happened to him in life, he would make the best of it. Are you that type of person? Because if you are not, then more than likely you will end up in what I call the "pity pot" corner. People go in that corner and cry "Poor me…poor me…poor me…poor me…poor me…."

How many of you would like to be a friend to a pity pot? Probably nobody. Then all we would hear from them would be "Poor me…poor me…nobody wants to be my friend."

Let's be honest, however. We are all human and from time to time we all end up in the pity pot corner. That's not the problem, though. The problem comes when you go there and stay. If that happens I guarantee you two things:

1. You are going to push everyone else away because no one wants to be with someone who is so negative all the time.

2. Not one darn thing in your circumstances will change. You will simply spend the rest of your days feeling sorry for yourself.

I don't know about you but that is not the kind of legacy I want to leave to my family and friends. I don't want my kids or grandchildren to remember me as someone who spent his remaining days feeling sorry for himself. The legacy I would rather leave is that although life may have thrown some curveballs at me through the aging process, I had the kind of attitude that I may not have liked all the things that happened, but I made the best of the situation.

Whether we are aware of it or not, we serve as role models for others. Others do notice how we handle the rough times of life and all the things that the aging process brings. What kind of role model do we want to leave as our legacy? The choice is up to us.

So, ask yourself this question: Am I the type of person who no matter what happens in life, I try to maintain a positive attitude? I may occasionally go into the pity pot corner but I am not going to stay there.

As the residents I had the privilege of serving always reminded me: Growing old is not for sissies. Our journeys go so much easier when we have a positive attitude packed in our suitcases to help us face whatever challenges lie ahead.

A Sense of Humor

In traveling this journey in life it is also important to have a healthy sense of humor packed away in our suitcase...to unpack it whenever we need to laugh at all the crazy things that happen as we walk the path of life. Let me give you some examples:

Have you ever walked into a room, scratched your head, and asked: Now why did I come in here?

Have you ever made a detailed grocery list and when you got to the store, you checked all your pockets and discovered the list was missing? When you got home later, there was the list grinning at you from the kitchen table.

I was doing laundry the other day and I had all my clothes in the washing machine except one black sock. I looked around the laundry room for several minutes until I looked down and discovered the missing black sock was still on my foot.

I have a hearing problem. Sometimes when someone says something to me, I'll hear one word instead of the actual one. I suspect many experience that as well. Let me give you but one example.

After a presentation I gave, a woman whom I hadn't seen for months came up to me and asked what I had been doing lately. When I told her that I was retired, she got this terrible expression of horror on her face and exclaimed, "You are retarded!" You see, she heard the word "retarded" for "retired". She had a hearing problem. I have a hearing problem. We could laugh about it. We didn't have to go into the pity pot corner and feel sorry for ourselves because we are losing our hearing.

One needs to have a sense of humor about life, especially as the aging process keeps coming at us. Because if we don't laugh every now and then, we'll end up crying all the time. I'm not talking about being childish or silly, but having a way of looking at the follies of life that aging brings that could be devastating if we didn't find some humor in them.

Allow me to share a joke with you told to me by a 91-year-old woman. The joke is about a woman called Gertrude who also was in her nineties. Gertrude just got home from the hospital. Any guesses as to why she was in the hospital. Stroke? Hip replacement? Pneumonia? Nope. She had a baby. That's right, you heard me...a baby.

The woman sharing this joke had a huge grin on her face as she continued:

Well, Gertrude wasn't home more than five minutes when there was a knock at her door. It was her neighbor. "Gertrude, I came over to see your baby." To which Gertrude replied, "Oh, good. Come in and have some coffee and cookies with me and I'll tell you all about it." The neighbor sat down on the couch in the living room and waited for Gertrude to get the cookies and coffee. They sat and had their treats and talked. Five minutes, ten minutes, fifteen, twenty minutes went by and finally the neighbor says, "Gertrude, I really have to get going. Can I see your baby?" "Well," Gertrude said with a perplexed look on her face, "You're going to have to wait until he cries because I can't remember where I put him down."

Remember, I told you that a 91-year-old woman shared that joke with me. What she was doing was inviting me into her world of memory loss…and asking me to laugh with her and not at her. That is an important distinction. It would be far different if someone in their 30's or 40's would tell that joke as a way of laughing at older people and their problems.

Let me share a couple of other stories that illustrate what I am talking about. These are true stories. After a presentation I made at a local church, an 85-year-old man came up to me and said, "You talk about having a sense of humor. Let me tell you about what happened when I went shopping with my daughter the other day. We were at a drugstore and my daughter was looking at some items in one of the aisles when I decided to go up to the pharmacist. I asked him if my prescription was ready. "What's your name?" he asked. I gave him my name and he said he would go back and check. After a few minutes, he came back and said with an apologetic tone, "I'm sorry, but we don't seem to have your prescription."

At that point I gave him my biggest grin and replied, "Good! That must mean I'm not sick!" I walked away wondering if the pharmacist knew I was just joshing with him.

On another occasion, after another presentation, I met a group of women out in the parking lot who had been in my seminar. One woman had a very tight smile when she looked at me, and I thought to myself, *Oh, oh, I'm in for something.*

She came up to me and said, "How can you say you should have a sense of humor when your car's been stolen."

"Are you sure?" I asked.

"Yes, I'm sure," she replied. She then pointed to an empty parking space ten feet away and cried, "Yes, I'm sure! I parked it right over there before the seminar. You don't see it, do you? It's gone."

Another woman came out and this woman ran up to her and said, "My car's been stolen!" The woman replied, "Are you sure you didn't park on the other side of the building."

"Yes, I'm sure!" she cried.

Another woman came out and this woman ran up to her and repeated her claim. "My car's been stolen! Do you think I should call the police?"

The woman just smiled and replied, "Dearie, don't you remember that you rode with me this morning."

It is important to have a sense of humor packed away in our suitcase as we make this journey because as I said, if we don't laugh sometimes, we'll end up crying all the time.

Meaning and Purpose

As a hobby, what do you collect? Stamps? Coins? Figurines? Plates? It seems like everyone at some time in their lives have collected one thing or another.

I met a man who collected left-handed monkey wrenches. When I asked how many he had, he said 16.

Another man, in his nineties, when asked what he collected, replied with a wry smile, "Dust."

One day I helped clean out a room of a gentleman who recently died. He had no family or friends. When we opened his closet door, there were stacks upon stacks of empty cereal boxes. Apparently, he collected them.

Another gentleman at the home, a retired engineer, loved to work on collages. He loved it so much that he spent seven days a week doing it. He loved it so much that we had a hard time getting him out for meals. And woe to the nurse who came in to give him his medication. She had to do it fast because, as he said, he had important work to do on his collages. He had no family to rely on for his supplies, but residents and staff supplied him with magazines so he would have an ample supply of pictures to use.

I watched him one afternoon. He would move a picture ½ of an inch and another one ¼ of an inch to make his masterpieces. I couldn't tell the difference but he sure could. He just loved doing his collages.

As we cleaned out his room we found a cardboard box, about 3 feet high, filled with collages he had finished. What do you think happened to them? Tossed out. That's right. They had no value other than to this gentleman. While he lived they gave him meaning and purpose in life.

And I would guess that the gentleman with the empty cereal boxes, his collection also gave him meaning and purpose.

Let me ask you to make a confession. (Remember confession is good for the soul.) How many of you ever wanted to be (or maybe were) hippies when you were younger? Perhaps none of you. Perhaps a few. Perhaps some of you wanted to be but were afraid. And perhaps some of you even right now wished you would have been a hippy.

Regardless of your feelings toward hippies, I think most of you knew what they were seeking...they were searching for the meaning and purpose of life. If you are near a window right now, what is out there? Trees? Buildings? A lake or river? Parking lot? Whatever. In a sense, hippies were looking out the window to search for the meaning of life...it had to be out there someplace.

Victor Frankel was a Jewish psychiatrist. As a young man, he was imprisoned in a Nazi concentration camp. During that time he tried to figure out why some people gave up and died while others survived. He came to the conclusion that for many of them who survived, they did so because they had some kind of meaning and purpose.

Released from the camp when the War ended, Frankel decided to enter the field of psychiatry. At some point in his professional life, he wrote a book called *Man's Search for Meaning*. One of the tenets of the book is that the meaning of life is not out there someplace, but rather within oneself. In other words, we give meaning and purpose to the things we do in life, whether it be collecting empty cereal boxes or making collages.

Always remember: we simply shouldn't let others decide what our meaning/purpose is. And please don't tell me that you're too old, too crippled, too worthless for anything anymore because I could tell you about a 98-year-old woman, bedridden and legally blind who spent her time on the third floor of the nursing home. Some might say how a 98-year-old woman, blind and bed ridden, can have any meaning or purpose in life anymore. And yet we would supply this woman with strips of red ribbon 8 to 10 inches long. Out of these ribbons, she would construct red roses. Don't ask me how she did it, but let me tell you they were beautiful works of art. She would give these roses to staff, other residents, and strangers. When she died we held a memorial service and many remembered her as the "Rose Lady". She had touched the lives of so many people. At age 98, bedridden, and legally blind, she still found meaning and purpose.

Be sure and reserve a spot in your suitcase for meaning and purpose. And don't ever forget, we have it within us, regardless of age and circumstance, to give meaning and purpose to life.

Ability to Love and Forgive

Aging does take a toll on us. I don't know about you, but my memory is not as good as it once was. I can't walk (and forget about running) as fast as I once did years ago. I have these strange spots appearing on my body (liver spots?). My skin is certainly not as smooth as it once was; more aches and pains; not as steady on my feet, etc., etc., etc.

You get the idea. We lose a lot of things as we age, but there are some things that the years cannot take away from us, and that is our ability to express love and forgiveness.

One of the greatest gifts we can give to our children, grandchildren, friends, is to remind them that the years have not diminished our love for them. I remember a new resident who just moved in. When I asked what I could do for her, she replied, "You're supposed to love me."

Forgiveness is also important to pack away in our suitcase. Our ancestors who travelled West in covered wagons learned a very important lesson in their journey that may be applied to us today. If you read any history of the wagon trains you will become aware that our ancestors realized that in order for them to complete their journeys, they needed to lighten their heavily loaded wagons. They tossed things out. By doing so, they could finish the journey.

Too many of us still have our lives loaded down with stuff that need to be tossed. What kind of stuff? Things like anger, resentment, bitterness, etc.

I recall being in a hospital as a patient years ago and listening to the man in the next bed tell the nurse, if his son came to see him, not to let him in, he didn't want to see him. Now, this man was dying. He also told me that he didn't even want his son to come to his funeral. I don't know whatever happened between him and his son to cause such a chasm, but it was just sad to hear.

Another woman told me that she had written to her sister to seek reconciliation over something that happened years ago...so long ago that she didn't remember what the original blowup was about. In the letter, she asked her sister to forgive her. Two weeks later, a reply came. Her sister wrote to tell her that she would never forgive her. When I asked her about that, she said that at least, she forgave her sister, and didn't have to carry that around anymore.

If you have any resentments, anger, etc. from the past, isn't it time to toss them, to lighten the load as you continue your journey? It's something to think about. Both love and forgiveness are items needed for the journey. Don't forget to pack them

Willingness to try New Things

Are you the type of person who is willing to try new and different things regardless of your age or circumstances? Or are you the type of person who believes that you simply can't teach new tricks to old dogs?

For my birthday one year, I received a set of oils and a blank canvas. I was in my forties at the time. Let me tell you that although I appreciated the gift, it scared me to death. Why? Because I was convinced that at my stage in life I couldn't learn something new or as complicated as oil painting. What if I screwed up the colors? What if the proportions were all wrong? What if...what if...what if?

So I put the oil paints and canvas in my closet, and shut the door. During the next year I would open up the closet door, take out a tube of oil, unscrew the cap, smell the oil, and then put the cap back on and put it back in the closet. I was too scared to try it. A year went by and I thought to myself *this is dumb*. So what if I mess up the colors. So what if everything is out of proportion? At least try it. So I did. My painting turned out amateurish, but do you know what: it added to my meaning and purpose. It wasn't the essence of my meaning and purpose, but it added.

When I began my work at the long-term facility (I was in my fifties now) I wanted to try something different in my approach to ministry. So I took up ventriloquism.

I remember my wife asking me one Christmas what I wanted for Christmas. When I replied "a home study course on ventriloquism," she eyed me for a moment and said with a twinkle in her eyes, "Boy, you are ready for the Home."

Well, I got the ventriloquism course and proceeded to take it step by step. It took me over four months to learn my voices and gather together some vent figures (they don't like to be referred to as "dummies"). I brought everything to my office but it took me another two weeks before I dared to venture out with one of my vent figures.

The reason? I thought to myself, What are people going to say when they see some guy in his fifties walking around with a doll?

Has he lost his mind? Has he slipped into his second childhood? Will they think it's childish, silly, or inappropriate? What if they see my lips move? What if they don't like my vent characters (I had five or six of them)? What if...what if...what if..?

After two weeks I said to myself that this is silly. So if they see my lips move…so if I'm not very good. At least try it. And do you know what? I took the chance and it went over pretty well.

It wasn't just fun and games, however. There was a serious side to it as well. There were some residents who wouldn't talk to staff but would talk to one of the vent figures. One woman who was dying asked not to see me as the chaplain or any of the other staff, but Ernie. Ernie was a furry dog who loved to hug and be hugged by the residents. This dying woman wanted to see Ernie. I brought him to see her. They talked, hugged, and said their good-byes. The next day the woman died.

A couple of weeks later one of the residents, an 85-year-old man, asked me if he could learn ventriloquism. I said sure and gave him the home study course, and off he went grinning like a kid with a new toy. I should tell you that this gentleman was dying of cancer at the time. Three weeks later he died, but he was willing at his age and in circumstances to learn something new. Are you that type of person? Are you willing to try something new regardless of your age or circumstances? Is there something right now that you have always wanted to try or do, but never got around to it? I tell you to go for it, whatever it may be. So what if you don't do a good job or you're not very good, even if you fall flat on your face, that is okay…it will add to your meaning and purpose.

I recall a woman in her 80's coming up to me to tell me what she is planning to do with her grandson on her upcoming 85th birthday. Can you guess? If you thought skydiving, you would be right. She said, "If President Bush can do it, so can I."

Another woman told me that she was planning to take a hot air balloon ride. She was only in her late 70's. Still, another woman told me that she was going to get herself something for her 65th birthday that she had always wanted but never got around to it. What is she planning? A tattoo! Now that may not be everyone's cup of tea but for this woman, it was her dream.

I will ask again: Is there something you always wanted to try or do but now are thinking it's too late…you're too old…you would not be able to do a good job…etc. I say go for it.

One final thought. If you are living someplace where there is an activity director on staff and he/she suggests something new…I hope you don't say, "I don't know. I have never done that before." Rather, I hope you would reply, "Just a minute. Let me get my suitcase. I've got my willingness to try new things packed in there."

An Anchor for the Storms of Life

Do you have a philosophy of life or a spiritual connection that can serve as an anchor when the storms of life come? Anybody who has lived for any length of time knows that life is full of storms. And the ones that come with aging seem to increase as the years go by.

There was a woman on the second floor of the nursing home who wanted to live to 100. She was 98 and determined to live to reach the century mark.

As a side note, I am curious. Would you, the reader, like to live to age 100? If you are like most people I have asked this question, your answer is no. Most groups I talk to only two or three people raised their hands when I ask how many would like to reach 100. Even when I spoke to an Optimist Club, only a few raised their hands. I couldn't compute that. I told them, "You are members of an Optimist Club, how come I didn't get more hands raised?"

The one group I spoke to where just about everybody raised their hands...can you guess? If you guessed a group of college-age kids, you would be right.

Anyway, this 98-year-old woman wanted to live to be a hundred. The only problem was that she had severe back problems and terrible arthritis. So that meant for the next two years she's going to live with pain every day. She was either in bed or if we got her up and put her into her wheelchair, she would be in pain. As the chaplain, I had to ask her how she balanced wanting to live for a couple more years knowing that every single day, she would be in pain. She was a woman of faith so I was curious to hear her answer. She said three words: "God suffers too." That was her anchor to get her by each day.

All of us need to have some kind of anchor as we travel this journey through life. It can be (as was the woman I just described) a spiritual anchor. It also could be a philosophy of life. One person told me that when a crisis arose in her life, she kept repeating to herself...this too shall pass...this too shall pass...this too shall pass.

Think about your journey. What or who is your anchor? And more importantly, is it packed securely in your suitcase?

The Moment of Truth

Have you ever experienced the moment of truth? You are probably scratching your head trying to figure out *what in the world is he asking*?

Let me clarify by asking it in a different way. When did you realize that you are not going to live forever?

I'm not talking intellectually…after all, we all know that this life does not go on and on. I am talking about when that fact smacks you in your gut.

I have known people who well into their 90's have never really had a moment of truth…and I have known kids who have. I will always remember this one fourteen-year-old boy who was facing major surgery and wasn't sure if he would survive it…he certainly had his moment of truth.

My moment of truth came when I was 33 years old. I was in the hospital undergoing tests for leukemia. Believe me, when you are waiting for the results of a test that could dramatically change your life, a lot of things go through your mind.

Now, I had been a minister for three years and had preached about hope, faith, etc. But for the first time in my life, I came to the thought that Chuck Tindell may not live forever. I realized that the walls of the house I was living in had a few cracks in them. For me, that was my moment of truth.

One Monday morning when I came to work at the senior facility I was working at, several staff came up to me and said, "We're so glad to see you."

You know, it's sort of nice to be greeted that way, it makes you feel sort of special. And then they said, "We thought you died."

I said, "What???"

To which they replied, "Yeah, we thought you died. Your obituary was in the paper."

One of the nurses brought me the paper and sure enough, in the obituary section was my name, Charles K Tindell. Married. 3 daughters.

Well, I am Charles E. Tindell. I have three children: 3 sons. After we straightened that out, I felt sort of good knowing that I would be missed.

About a week later I get a phone call from Jim, a friend of mine that I hadn't seen in thirty years. The conversation went as follows:

Jim: "I went to your funeral."

Me: "Oh? Is that right? And how did I look?"

Jim: "You didn't look like yourself."

Me: "Jim, at what point did you realize it wasn't me?"

Jim: "About halfway through the eulogy. I couldn't get up and walk out, however, because that would have been tacky."

The above is a true story. I keep that obituary in my wallet to remind me, not in a morbid way, of how fragile life can be. It reminds me to celebrate each day, each hour, and each moment. I'm not talking about looking at life through rose-colored glasses, but learning to appreciate the time I still have left to experience. Does that mean that everything that happens to us in life is going to be to our liking? Of course not. Let's not be naïve.

But because we have a positive attitude, a sense of humor, meaning, and purpose in life, a commitment to love and to forgive, a willingness to try new things, and an anchor for the storms when they come, we are better equipped to deal with life as we continue to travel our journey.

So check your suitcases to see what you have packed for the journey. Believe me; it makes all the difference in the world having the right things for the road ahead.

One final thought: If you make friends with the aging process, you'll find that the journey will be much easier.

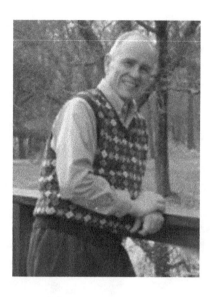

Charles Tindell's writing career began one hot July day in 1995 while sitting in a canoe in the Boundary Waters Canoe Area in northern Minnesota. His first book *Seeing Beyond the Wrinkles* is the recipient of the National Mature Media's coveted GOLD AWARD designating it among "The Best in Educational Material for Older Adults." His second book *The Enduring Human Spirit* is the recipient of the National Mature Media's Silver Award, symbolizing that the work is among the best of the best.

He and his wife, Carol, have three sons, four grandchildren, and two cats. Oil painting, ventriloquism, baking bread, canoeing, jigsaw puzzles, collecting hour glasses, and writing are among his interests. He serves as a volunteer police chaplain for his community. He also has had the privilege of speaking around the country on the subjects *Spirituality and Aging* as well as *The Courage to Be*. He has also written a novel titled *Grandpa's*

Legacy. His latest book, *Life's Journey: What's in your suitcase?* is based on his many years as a Pastor helping people with their own life's journeys.

Charles just completed the eighth mystery in *the* MAC Detective Agency series featuring Howie Cummins and his partners, Adam Trexler and Mick Brunner—*This Angel Loves Mysteries.* The previous mysteries in the series are: *This Angel Has No Wings, This Angel Doesn't like Chocolate, This Angel's Halo Is Crooked, This Angel Isn't Funny, This Angel Has Blue Eyes, This Angel is Going Down, and This Angel Doesn't Play Nice.*

CPSIA information can be obtained
at www.ICGtesting.com
Printed in the USA
JSHW020321060223
37325JS00001B/45